Air Fried Seafood Specialties

Tasty Keto Air Fried Seafood Dishes

Lucy Grant

Table of Contents

Introduction

What's the difference between an air fryer and deep fryer? Air fryers bake food at a high temperature with a high-powered fan, while deep fryers cook food in a vat of oil that has been heated up to a specific temperature. Both cook food quickly, but an air fryer requires practically zero preheat time while a deep fryer can take upwards of 10 minutes. Air fryers also require little to no oil and deep fryers require a lot that absorb into the food. Food comes out crispy and juicy in both appliances, but don't taste the same, usually because deep fried foods are coated in batter that cook differently in an air fryer vs a deep fryer. Battered foods needs to be sprayed with oil before cooking in an air fryer to help them color and get crispy, while the hot oil soaks into the batter in a deep fryer. Flour-based batters and wet batters don't cook well in an air fryer, but they come out very well in a deep fryer.

The ketogenic diet is one such example. The diet calls for a very small number of carbs to be eaten. This means food such as rice, pasta, and other starchy vegetables like potatoes are off the menu. Even relaxed versions of the keto diet minimize carbs to a large extent and this compromises the goals of many dieters. They end up having to exert large amounts of willpower to follow the diet. This doesn't do them any favors since willpower is like a muscle. At some point, it tires and this is when the dieter goes right back to their old pattern of eating. I have personal experience with this. In terms of health benefits, the keto diet offers the most. The reduction of carbs forces your body to mobilize fat and this results in automatic fat loss and better health.

Feel free to mix and match the recipes you see in here and play around with them. Eating is supposed to be fun! Unfortunately, we've associated fun eating with unhealthy food. This doesn't have to be the case. The air fryer, combined with the Mediterranean diet, will make your mealtimes fun-filled again and full of taste. There's no grease and messy cleanups to deal with anymore. Are you excited yet?

You should be! You're about to embark on a journey full of air fried goodness!

Old Bay Calamari

Prep + Cook Time: 20 minutes + Marinating Time

3 Servings

INGREDIENTS

1 cup beer

1 pound squid, cleaned and cut into rings

1 cup all-purpose flour

2 eggs

1/2 cup cornstarch

Sea salt, to taste

1/2 teaspoon ground black pepper

1 tablespoon Old Bay seasoning

DIRECTIONS

Add the beer and squid in a glass bowl, cover and let it sit in your refrigerator for 1 hour.

Preheat your Air Fryer to 390 degrees F.

Rinse the squid and pat it dry.

Place the flour in a shallow bowl.

In another bowl, whisk the eggs.

Add the cornstarch and seasonings to a third shallow bowl.

Dredge the calamari in the flour.

Then, dip them into the egg mixture; finally, coat them with the cornstarch on all sided.

Arrange them in the cooking basket.

Spritz with cooking oil and cook for 9 to 12 minutes, depending on the desired level of doneness.

Work in batches.

Serve warm with your favorite dipping sauce.

Enjoy!

Grilled Tilapia with Portobello Mushrooms

Prep + Cook Time: 20 minutes 2

Servings

INGREDIENTS

2 tilapia fillets

1 tablespoon avocado oil

1/2 teaspoon red pepper flakes, crushed

1/2 teaspoon dried sage, crushed

1/4 teaspoon lemon pepper

1/2 teaspoon sea salt

1 teaspoon dried parsley flakes

4 medium-sized Portobello mushrooms

A few drizzles of liquid smoke

DIRECTIONS

Toss all ingredients in a mixing bowl; except for the mushrooms.

Transfer the tilapia fillets to a lightly greased grill pan.

Preheat your Air Fryer to 400 degrees F and cook the tilapia fillets for 5 minutes.

Now, turn the fillets over and add the Portobello mushrooms.

Continue to cook for 5 minutes longer or until mushrooms are tender and the fish is opaque.

Serve immediately.

Enjoy!

Crunchy Topped Fish Bake

Prep + Cook Time: 20 minutes

4 Servings

INGREDIENTS

1 tablespoon butter, melted

1 medium-sized leek, thinly sliced

1 tablespoon chicken stock

1 tablespoon dry white wine

1 pound tuna

1/2 teaspoon red pepper flakes, crushed

Sea salt and ground black pepper, to taste

1/2 teaspoon dried rosemary

1/2 teaspoon dried basil

1/2 teaspoon dried thyme

2 ripe tomatoes, pureed

1/4 cup breadcrumbs

1/4 cup Parmesan cheese, grated

DIRECTIONS

Melt 1/2 tablespoon of butter in a sauté pan over medium-high heat.

Now, cook the leek and garlic until tender and aromatic.

Add the stock and wine to deglaze the pan.

Preheat your Air Fryer to 370 degrees F.

Grease a casserole dish with the remaining 1/2 tablespoon of melted butter.

Place the fish in the casserole dish.

Add the seasonings.

Top with the sautéed leek mixture.

Add the tomato puree.

Cook for 10 minutes in the preheated Air Fryer.

Top with the breadcrumbs and cheese; cook an additional 7 minutes until the crumbs are golden.

Serve and enjoy!

Beer Battered Fish with Honey Tartar Sauce

Prep + Cook Time: 20 minutes

2 Servings

INGREDIENTS

1/2 pound hoki fillets

Sea salt and black pepper, to taste

1/2 cup flour

1 egg

1 teaspoon paprika

1 12-ounce bottle beer

1/4 cup mayonnaise

1/2 teaspoon honey

1 tablespoon fresh lemon juice

1 teaspoon Dijon mustard

1 teaspoon sweet pickle relish

DIRECTIONS

Rinse the hoki fillets and pat dry.

Combine the flour, egg and paprika in a bowl.

Gradually pour in beer until a batter is formed.

Dip the fish fillets into the batter; then, transfer to the lightly greased cooking basket.

Cook in the preheated Air Fryer at 380 degrees F for 12 minutes.

In the meantime, whisk the remaining ingredients to make the sauce.

Place in the refrigerator until ready to serve.

Enjoy!

Snapper with Coconut Milk Sauce

Prep + Cook Time: 20 minutes + Marinating Time

2 Servings

INGREDIENTS

1/2 cup full-fat coconut milk

2 tablespoons lemon juice

1 teaspoon fresh ginger, grated

2 snapper fillets

1 tablespoon olive oil

1 tablespoon cornstarch

Salt and white pepper, to taste

DIRECTIONS

Place the milk, lemon juice, and ginger in a glass bowl; add fish and let it marinate for 1 hour.

Removed the fish from the milk mixture and place in the Air Fryer basket.

Drizzle olive oil all over the fish fillets.

Cook in the preheated Air Fryer at 390 degrees F for 15 minutes.

Meanwhile, heat the milk mixture over medium-high heat; bring to a rapid boil, stirring continuously.

Reduce to simmer and add the cornstarch, salt, and pepper; continue to cook 12 minutes more.

Spoon the sauce over the warm snapper fillets and serve immediately.

Moroccan Harissa Shrimp

Prep + Cook Time: 10 minutes

3 Servings

INGREDIENTS

1pound breaded shrimp, frozen

1 teaspoon extra-virgin olive oil

Sea salt and ground black pepper, to taste

1 teaspoon coriander seeds

1 teaspoon caraway seeds

1 teaspoon crushed red pepper

1 teaspoon fres garlic, minced

DIRECTIONS

Toss the breaded shrimp with olive oil and transfer to the Air Fryer cooking basket.

Cook in the preheated Air Fryer at 400 degrees F for 5 minutes; shake the basket and cook an additional 4 minutes.

Meanwhile, mix the remaining ingredients until well combined.

Taste and adjust seasonings.

Toss the warm shrimp with the harissa sauce and serve immediately.

Enjoy!

Anchovy and Cheese Wontons

Prep + Cook Time: 15 minutes

2 Servings

INGREDIENTS

½ pound anchovies

½ cup cheddar cheese, grated

1 cup fresh spinach

2 tablespoons scallions, minced

1 teaspoon garlic, minced

1 tablespoon Shoyu sauce

Himalayan salt and ground black pepper, to taste

½ pound wonton wrappers

1 teaspoon sesame oil

DIRECTIONS

Mash the anchovies and mix with the cheese, spinach, scallions, garlic and Shoyu sauce; season with salt and black pepper and mix to combine well.

Fill your wontons with 1 tablespoon of the filling mixture and fold into triangle shape; brush the side with a bit of oil and water to seal the edges.

Cook in your Air Fryer at 390 degrees F for 10 minutes, flipping the wontons for even cooking.

Enjoy!

Seed-Crusted Codfish Fillets

Prep + Cook Time: 15 minutes

2 Servings

INGREDIENTS

2 codfish fillets

1 teaspoon sesame oil

Sea salt and black pepper, to taste

1 teaspoon sesame seeds

1 tablespoon chia seeds

DIRECTIONS

Start by preheating your Air Fryer to 380 degrees F.

Add the sesame oil, salt, black pepper, sesame seeds and chia seeds to a rimmed plate.

Coat the top of the codfish with the seed mixture, pressing it down to adhere.

Lower the codfish fillets, seed side down, into the cooking basket and cook for 6 minutes.

Turn the fish fillets over and cook for a further 6 minutes.

Serve warm and enjoy!

Tuna Steaks with Pearl Onions

Prep + Cook Time: 20 minutes

4 Servings

INGREDIENTS

4 tuna steaks

1 pound pearl onions

4 teaspoons olive oil

1 teaspoon dried rosemary

1 teaspoon dried marjoram

1 tablespoon cayenne pepper

1/2 teaspoon sea salt

1/2 teaspoon black pepper, preferably freshly cracked

1 lemon, sliced

DIRECTIONS

Place the tuna steaks in the lightly greased cooking basket.

Top with the pearl onions; add the olive oil, rosemary, marjoram, cayenne pepper, salt, and black pepper.

Bake in the preheated Air Fryer at 400 degrees F for 9 to 10 minutes.

Work in two batches.

Serve warm with lemon slices and enjoy!

English-Style Flounder Fillets

Prep + Cook Time: 20 minutes

2 Servings

INGREDIENTS

2 flounder fillets

1/4 cup all-purpose flour

1 egg

1/2 teaspoon Worcestershire sauce

1/2 cup bread crumbs

1/2 teaspoon lemon pepper

1/2 teaspoon coarse sea salt

1/4 teaspoon chili powder

DIRECTIONS

Rinse and pat dry the flounder fillets.

Place the flour in a large pan.

Whisk the egg and Worcestershire sauce in a shallow bowl.

In a separate bowl, mix the bread crumbs with the lemon pepper, salt, and chili powder.

Dredge the fillets in the flour, shaking off the excess.

Then, dip them into the egg mixture.

Lastly, coat the fish fillets with the breadcrumb mixture until they are coated on all sides.

Spritz with cooking spray and transfer to the Air Fryer basket.

Cook at 390 degrees for 7 minutes.

Turn them over, spritz with cooking spray on the other side, and cook another 5 minutes.

Serve and enjoy!

Quick-Fix Seafood Breakfast

Prep + Cook Time: 30 minutes

2 Servings

INGREDIENTS

1 tablespoon olive oil

2 garlic cloves, minced

1 small yellow onion, chopped

1/4 pound tilapia pieces

1/4 pound rockfish pieces

1/2 teaspoon dried basil

Salt and white pepper, to taste

4 eggs, lightly beaten

1 tablespoon dry sherry

4 tablespoons cheese, shredded

DIRECTIONS

Start by preheating your Air Fryer to 350 degrees F; add the olive oil to a baking pan.

Once hot, cook the garlic and onion for 2 minutes or until fragrant.

Add the fish, basil, salt, and pepper.

In a mixing dish, thoroughly combine the eggs with sherry and cheese.

Pour the mixture into the baking pan.

Cook at 360 degrees F approximately 20 minutes.

Serve and enjoy!

Grilled Hake with Garlic Sauce

Prep + Cook Time: 20 minutes

3 Servings

INGREDIENTS

3 hake fillets

6 tablespoons mayonnaise

1 teaspoon Dijon mustard

1 tablespoon fresh lime juice

1 cup panko crumbs

Salt, to taste

1/4 teaspoon ground black pepper, or more to taste

Garlic Sauce:

1/4 cup Greek-style yogurt

2 tablespoons olive oil

2 cloves garlic, minced

1/2 teaspoon tarragon leaves, minced

DIRECTIONS

Pat dry the hake fillets with a kitchen towel.

In a shallow bowl, whisk together the mayo, mustard, and lime juice.

In another shallow bowl, thoroughly combine the panko crumbs with salt, and black pepper.

Spritz the Air Fryer grill pan with non-stick cooking spray.

Grill in the preheated Air Fry at 395 degrees F for 10 minutes, flipping halfway through the cooking time.

Serve immediately.

Buttermilk Tuna fillets

Prep + Cook Time: 50 minutes

3 Servings

INGREDIENTS

1 pound tuna fillets

1/2 cup buttermilk

1/2 cup tortilla chips, crushed

1/4 cup parmesan cheese, grated

1/4 cup cassava flour

Salt and ground black pepper, to taste

1 teaspoon mustard seeds

1 teaspoon paprika

1 teaspoon garlic powder

1/2 teaspoon onion powder

DIRECTIONS

Place the tuna fillets and buttermilk in a bowl; cover and let it sit for 30 minutes.

In a shallow bowl, thoroughly combine the remaining ingredients; mix until well combined.

Dip the tuna fillets in the parmesan mixture until they are covered on all sides.

Cook in the preheated Air Fryer at 380 degrees F for 12 minutes, turning halfway through the cooking time.

Serve and enjoy!

King Prawns with Lemon Butter Sauce

Prep + Cook Time: 15 minutes

4 Servings

INGREDIENTS

King Prawns:

1 ½ pounds king prawns, peeled and deveined

2 cloves garlic, minced

1/2 cup Pecorino Romano cheese, grated

Sea salt and ground white pepper, to your liking

1/2 teaspoon onion powder

1 teaspoon garlic powder

1 teaspoon mustard seeds

2 tablespoons olive oil

Sauce:

2 tablespoons butter

2 tablespoons fresh lemon juice

1/2 teaspoon Worcestershire sauce

1/4 teaspoon ground black pepper

DIRECTIONS

In a plastic closeable bag, thoroughly combine all ingredients for the king prawns; shake to combine well.

Transfer the coated king prawns to the lightly greased Air Fryer basket.

Cook in the preheated Air Fryer at 390 degrees for 6 minutes, shaking the basket halfway through.

Work in batches.

In the meantime, heat a small saucepan over a moderate flame; melt the butter and add the remaining ingredients.

Turn the temperature to low and whisk for 2 to 3 minutes until thoroughly heated.

Spoon the sauce onto the warm king prawns.

Serve and enjoy!

Sea Bass with French Sauce Tartare

Prep + Cook Time: 15 minutes

2 Servings

INGREDIENTS

1 tablespoon olive oil

2 sea bass fillets

Sauce:

1/2 cup mayonnaise

1 tablespoon capers, drained and chopped

1 tablespoon gherkins, drained and chopped

2 tablespoons scallions, finely chopped

2 tablespoons lemon juice

DIRECTIONS

Start by preheating your Air Fryer to 395 degrees F.

Drizzle olive oil all over the fish fillets.

Cook the sea bass in the preheated Air Fryer for 10 minutes, flipping them halfway through the cooking time.

Meanwhile, make the sauce by whisking the remaining ingredients until everything is well incorporated.

Place in the refrigerator until ready to serve.

Enjoy!

Rosemary-Infused Butter Scallops

Prep + Cook Time: 1 hour 10 minutes

4 Servings

INGREDIENTS

2 pounds sea scallops

1/2 cup beer

4 tablespoons butter

2 sprigs rosemary, only leaves

Sea salt and freshly cracked black pepper, to taste

DIRECTIONS

In a ceramic dish, mix the sea scallops with beer; let it marinate for 1 hour.

Meanwhile, preheat your Air Fryer to 400 degrees F.

Melt the butter and add the rosemary leaves.

Stir for a few minutes.

Discard the marinade and transfer the sea scallops to the Air Fryer basket.

Season with salt and black pepper.

Cook the scallops in the preheated Air Fryer for 7 minutes, shaking the basket halfway through the cooking time.

Work in batches.

Greek Sardeles Psites

Prep + Cook Time: 40 minutes

2 Servings

INGREDIENTS

4 sardines, cleaned

1/4 cup all-purpose flour

Sea salt and ground black pepper, to taste

4 tablespoons extra-virgin olive oil

1/2 red onion, chopped

1/2 teaspoon fresh garlic, minced

1/4 cup sweet white wine

1 tablespoon fresh coriander, minced

1/4 cup baby capers, drained

1 tomato, crushed

1/4 teaspoon chili paper flakes

DIRECTIONS

Coat your sardines with all-purpose flour until well coated on all sides.

Season your sardines with salt and black pepper and arrange them in the cooking basket.

Cook in your Air Fryer at 325 degrees F for 35 to 40 minutes until the skin is crispy.

Meanwhile, heat olive oil in a frying pan over a moderate flame.

Now, sauté the onion and garlic for 4 to 5 minutes or until tender and aromatic.

Stir in the remaining ingredients, cover and let it simmer, for about 15 minutes or until the sauce has thickened and reduced.

Spoon the sauce over the warm sardines and serve immediately.

Enjoy!

Halibut Steak with Cremini Mushrooms

Prep + Cook Time: 15 minutes

3 Servings

INGREDIENTS

1 pound halibut steak

1 teaspoon olive oil

Sea salt and ground black pepper, to taste

7 ounces Cremini mushrooms

1 teaspoon butter, melted

1/4 teaspoon onion powder

1/4 teaspoon garlic powder

1/2 teaspoon rosemary

1/2 teaspoon basil

1/2 teaspoon oregano

DIRECTIONS

Toss the halibut steak with olive oil, salt and black pepper and transfer to the Air Fryer cooking basket.

Toss the Cremini mushrooms with the other ingredients until well coated on all sides.

Cook the halibut steak at 400 degrees F for 5 minutes.

Turn the halibut steak over and top with mushrooms.

Continue to cook an additional 5 minutes or until the mushrooms are fragrant.

Serve warm and enjoy!

Haddock Steaks with Decadent Mango Salsa

Prep + Cook Time: 15 minutes

2 Servings

INGREDIENTS

2 haddock steaks

1 teaspoon butter, melted

1 tablespoon white wine

Sea salt and ground black pepper, to taste

Mango salsa:

1/2 mango, diced

1/4 cup red onion, chopped

1 chili pepper, deveined and minced

1 teaspoon cilantro, chopped

2 tablespoons fresh lemon juice

DIRECTIONS

Toss the haddock with butter, wine, salt and black pepper.

Cook the haddock in your Air Fryer at 400 degrees F for 5 minutes.

Flip the haddock and cook on the other side for 5 minutes more.

Meanwhile, make the mango salsa by mixing all ingredients.

Serve the warm haddock with the chilled mango salsa and enjoy!

Halibut Steak with Zoodles and Lemon

Prep + Cook Time: 15 minutes

3 Servings

INGREDIENTS

1 pound halibut steak, cut into

3 pieces

1 garlic clove, halved

1 teaspoon avocado oil

Sea salt and black pepper, to taste

1 pound zucchini, julienned

1/2 teaspoon onion powder

1/2 teaspoon granulated garlic

1 tablespoon fresh parsley, minced

1 teaspoon sage, minced

1 lemon, sliced

DIRECTIONS

Rub the halibut steaks with garlic and toss with avocado oil, salt and black pepper; then, transfer the halibut steaks to the Air Fryer cooking basket.

Cook the halibut steak at 400 degrees F for 5 minutes.

Turn the halibut steak over and continue to cook an additional 5 minutes or until it flakes easily when tested with a fork.

Meanwhile, spritz a wok with a nonstick spray; heat the wok over medium-high heat.

Once hot, stir fry the zucchini noodles along with the onion powder and granulated garlic; cook for 2 to 3 minutes or until just tender.

Top your zoodles with the parsley and sage and stir to combine.

Serve the hot zoodles with the halibut steaks and lemon slices.

Enjoy!

Saucy Garam Masala Fish

Prep + Cook Time: 25 minutes

2 Servings

INGREDIENTS

2 teaspoons olive oil

1/4 cup coconut milk

1/2 teaspoon cayenne pepper

1 teaspoon Garam masala

1/4 teaspoon Kala namak

Indian black salt

1/2 teaspoon fresh ginger, grated

1 garlic clove, minced

2 catfish fillets

1/4 cup coriander, roughly chopped

DIRECTIONS

Preheat your Air Fryer to 390 degrees F.

Then, spritz the baking dish with a nonstick cooking spray.

In a mixing bowl, whisk the olive oil, milk, cayenne pepper, Garam masala, Kala namak, ginger, and garlic.

Coat the catfish fillets with the Garam masala mixture.

Cook the catfish fillets in the preheated Air Fryer approximately 18 minutes, turning over halfway through the cooking time.

Garnish with fresh coriander and serve over hot noodles if desired.

Enjoy!

Old Bay Shrimp

Preparation Time: 10 minutes

Cooking Time: 10 minutes

Serve: 4

Ingredients:

12 oz shrimp, peeled

3/25 oz pork rind, crushed

1 1/2 tsp old bay seasoning

1/4 cup mayonnaise

Directions:

In a shallow bowl, mix together crushed pork rind and old bay seasoning.

Add shrimp and mayonnaise into the mixing bowl and toss well.

Place the cooking tray in the air fryer basket.

Select Air Fry mode.

Set time to 10 minutes and temperature 380 F then press START.

The air fryer display will prompt you to ADD FOOD once the temperature is reached then coat shrimp with crushed pork rind and place in the air fryer basket.

Serve and enjoy.

Garlic Butter Fish Fillets

Preparation Time: 10 minutes

Cooking Time: 10 minutes

Serve: 2

Ingredients:

2 salmon fillets

1/4 tsp dried parsley

1 tsp garlic, minced

2 tbsp butter, melted

Pepper

Salt

Directions:

In a small bowl, mix together melted butter, garlic, and parsley.

Season fish fillets with pepper and salt and brush with melted butter mixture.

Place the cooking tray in the air fryer basket.

Select Air Fry mode.

Set time to 10 minutes and temperature 360 F then press START.

The air fryer display will prompt you to ADD FOOD once the temperature is reached then place fish fillets skin side down in the air fryer basket.

Serve and enjoy.

Flavorful Tuna Steaks

Preparation Time: 10 minutes

Cooking Time: 4 minutes

Serve: 2

Ingredients:

12 tuna steaks, skinless and boneless

1/2 tsp rice vinegar

1 tsp sesame oil

1 tsp ginger, grated

4 tbsp soy sauce

Directions:

Add tuna steaks and remaining ingredients in the zip-lock bag.

Seal bag and place in the refrigerator for 30 minutes.

Select Air Fry mode.

Set time to 4 minutes and temperature 380 F then press START.

The air fryer display will prompt you to ADD FOOD once the temperature is reached then place marinated tuna steaks in the air fryer basket.

Serve and enjoy.

Baked Parmesan Tilapia

Preparation Time: 10 minutes

Cooking Time: 10 minutes

Serve: 4

Ingredients:

2 lbs tilapia

1/4 tsp paprika

1/4 tsp dried basil

2 garlic cloves, minced

1 tsp dried parsley

1 tbsp butter, softened

2 tbsp fresh lemon juice

1/4 cup mayonnaise

1/2 cup parmesan cheese, grated

1/2 tsp salt

Directions:

In a small bowl, mix together parmesan cheese, mayonnaise, lemon juice, butter, parsley, garlic, basil, paprika, and salt.

Place the cooking tray in the air fryer basket.

Line air fryer basket with parchment paper.

Select Bake mode.

Set time to 10 minutes and temperature 400 F then press START.

The air fryer display will prompt you to ADD FOOD once the temperature is reached then place fish fillets in the air fryer basket and spread the parmesan mixture on top of each fish fillet.

Serve and enjoy.

Bagel Crust Fish Fillets

Preparation Time: 10 minutes

Cooking Time: 10 minutes

Serve: 4

Ingredients:

4 white fish fillets

1 tbsp mayonnaise

1 tsp lemon pepper seasoning

2 tbsp almond flour

1/4 cup bagel seasoning

Directions:

In a small bowl, mix together bagel seasoning, almond flour, and lemon pepper seasoning.

Brush mayonnaise over fish fillets. Sprinkle seasoning mixture over fish fillets.

Place the cooking tray in the air fryer basket.

Line air fryer basket with parchment paper.

Select Bake mode.

Set time to 10 minutes and temperature 400 F then press START.

The air fryer display will prompt you to ADD FOOD once the temperature is reached then place fish fillets in the air fryer basket.

Serve and enjoy.

Baked Salmon Patties

Preparation Time: 10 minutes

Cooking Time: 20 minutes

Serve: 4

Ingredients:

2 eggs, lightly beaten

12 oz can salmon, skinless, boneless, and drained

1/2 cup almond flour

1/2 tsp pepper

1 tbsp Dijon mustard

1 tsp garlic powder

2 tbsp fresh parsley, chopped

1/2 cup celery, diced

1/2 cup bell pepper, diced

1/2 cup onion, diced

Directions:

Add salmon and remaining ingredients into the mixing bowl and mix until well combined.

Make 8 equal shapes of patties from the mixture.

Place the cooking tray in the air fryer basket.

Line air fryer basket with parchment paper.

Select Bake mode.

Set time to 20 minutes and temperature 400 F then press START.

The air fryer display will prompt you to ADD FOOD once the temperature is reached then place patties in the air fryer basket.

Turn patties halfway through. Serve and enjoy.

Pesto Scallops

Preparation Time: 10 minutes

Cooking Time: 7 minutes

Serve: 4

Ingredients:

1 lb sea scallops

2 tsp garlic, minced

3 tbsp heavy cream

1/4 cup basil pesto

1 tbsp olive oil

1/2 tsp pepper

1 tsp salt

Directions:

In a small pan, mix together oil, cream, garlic, pesto, pepper, and salt, and simmer for 2-3 minutes.

Select Air Fry mode.

Set time to 5 minutes and temperature 320 F then press START. The air fryer display will prompt you to ADD FOOD once the temperature is reached then add scallops in the air fryer basket.

Turn scallops and after 3 minutes.

Transfer scallops into the mixing bowl.

Pour pesto sauce over scallops and serve.

Juicy Baked Halibut

Preparation Time: 10 minutes

Cooking Time: 12 minutes

Serve: 4

Ingredients:

1 lb halibut fillets

1/4 tsp garlic powder

1/4 tsp paprika

1/4 tsp pepper

1/4 cup olive oil

1 lemon juice

1/2 tsp salt

Directions:

In a small bowl, mix together olive oil, lemon juice, pepper, paprika, garlic powder, and salt.

Brush olive oil mixture over fish fillets.

Place the cooking tray in the air fryer basket.

Line air fryer basket with parchment paper.

Select Bake mode.

Set time to 12 minutes and temperature 400 F then press START.

The air fryer display will prompt you to ADD FOOD once the temperature is reached then place fish fillets in the air fryer basket.

Serve and enjoy.

Simple Salmon Patties

Preparation Time: 10 minutes

Cooking Time: 14 minutes

Serve: 4

Ingredients:

2 eggs, lightly beaten

2 oz salmon, cooked and flaked

1/4 tsp paprika

1/8 tsp pepper

1/3 cup parsley, chopped

2 garlic cloves, minced

1/4 cup onion, diced

2/3 cup almond flour

Pinch of salt

Directions:

Add all ingredients into the mixing bowl and mix until well combined.

Make the equal shape of patties from the mixture.

Place the cooking tray in the air fryer basket.

Line air fryer basket with parchment paper.

Select Air Fry mode.

Set time to 14 minutes and temperature 380 F then press START.

The air fryer display will prompt you to ADD FOOD once the temperature is reached then place patties in the air fryer basket.

Turn patties halfway through.

Serve and enjoy.

Baked Mahi Mahi

Preparation Time: 10 minutes

Cooking Time: 30 minutes

Serve: 4

Ingredients:

4 Mahi Mahi fillets

1 tsp onion powder

1 tsp garlic powder

1 tsp turmeric

1 tbsp dried basil

1 tsp pepper

1 tsp salt

Directions:

In a small bowl, mix together onion powder, garlic powder, turmeric, basil, pepper, and salt.

Season fish fillets with spice mixture.

Place the cooking tray in the air fryer basket.

Line air fryer basket with parchment paper.

Select Bake mode.

Set time to 30 minutes and temperature 350 F then press START.

The air fryer display will prompt you to ADD FOOD once the temperature is reached then place the fish fillet in the air fryer basket.

Serve and enjoy.

Parmesan Cod

Preparation Time: 10 minutes

Cooking Time: 15 minutes

Serve: 4

Ingredients:

4 cod fillets

1 tbsp olive oil

1 tbsp parsley, chopped

2 tsp paprika

3/4 cup parmesan cheese, grated

1/4 tsp sea salt

Directions:

In a shallow dish, mix together parmesan cheese, paprika, parsley, and salt.

Brush fish fillets with oil and coat with cheese mixture.

Place the cooking tray in the air fryer basket.

Line air fryer basket with parchment paper.

Select Bake mode.

Set time to 15 minutes and temperature 400 F then press START.

The air fryer display will prompt you to ADD FOOD once the temperature is reached then place the fish fillet in the air fryer basket.

Serve and enjoy.

Baked Mayo Cod

Preparation Time: 10 minutes

Cooking Time: 10 minutes

Serve: 4

Ingredients:

4 cod fillets

1/2 cup almond flour

1 tbsp parsley, chopped

1/2 tsp old bay seasoning

1/2 tsp lemon zest

1 tbsp lemon juice

1/4 cup parmesan cheese, grated

1/4 cup onion, minced

2 tbsp butter, melted

1/3 cup mayonnaise

Directions:

In a bowl, mix together mayonnaise, butter, onion, cheese, lemon juice, lemon zest, old bay seasoning, and parsley.

Spread mayonnaise mixture on top of fish fillets.

Sprinkle with almond flour.

Place the cooking tray in the air fryer basket.

Line air fryer basket with parchment paper.

Select Bake mode.

Set time to 10 minutes and temperature 400 F then press START.

The air fryer display will prompt you to ADD FOOD once the temperature is reached then place the fish fillet in the air fryer basket.

Serve and enjoy.

Lemon Pepper Tilapia

Preparation Time: 10 minutes

Cooking Time: 15 minutes

Serve: 4

Ingredients:

4 tilapia fillets, thawed

4 tbsp lemon pepper seasoning

Directions:

Spray fish fillets with cooking spray.

Sprinkle lemon pepper seasoning over fish fillets.

Place the cooking tray in the air fryer basket.

Line air fryer basket with parchment paper.

Select Bake mode.

Set time to 15 minutes and temperature 350 F then press START.

The air fryer display will prompt you to ADD FOOD once the temperature is reached then place the fish fillet in the air fryer basket.

Serve and enjoy.

Cajun Salmon Cakes

Preparation Time: 10 minutes

Cooking Time: 15 minutes

Serve: 4

Ingredients:

2 eggs, lightly beaten

12 oz can salmon, boneless & skinless

3/4 cup almond flour

2 1/2 tsp Cajun seasoning

1/2 onion, chopped

1/2 bell pepper, chopped

2 tbsp mayonnaise

Pepper

Salt

Directions:

Add all ingredients into the mixing bowl and mix until well combined.

Make 8 equal shapes of patties from the mixture.

Place the cooking tray in the air fryer basket.

Line air fryer basket with parchment paper.

Select Bake mode.

Set time to 10 minutes and temperature 375 F then press START.

The air fryer display will prompt you to ADD FOOD once the temperature is reached then add patties in the air fryer basket.

Broil patties for 5 minutes.

Serve and enjoy.

Old Bay Shrimp

Preparation Time: 10 minutes

Cooking Time: 10 minutes

Serve: 4

Ingredients:

1 lb shrimp, peeled & deveined

1 tbsp old bay seasoning

1/2 tbsp garlic, minced

1/2 tbsp lemon juice

1/2 tbsp olive oil

Directions:

Add shrimp and remaining ingredients into the mixing bowl and toss well.

Place the cooking tray in the air fryer basket.

Select Air Fry mode.

Set time to 10 minutes and temperature 390 F then press START.

The air fryer display will prompt you to ADD FOOD once the temperature is reached then add shrimp in the air fryer basket.

Serve and enjoy.

Healthy Lemon Pepper Shrimp

Preparation Time: 10 minutes

Cooking Time: 8 minutes

Serve: 2

Ingredients:

12 oz shrimp, peeled and deveined

1 lemon, sliced

1/4 tsp garlic powder

1/4 tsp paprika

1 tsp lemon pepper

1 lemon juice

1/2 tbsp olive oil

Directions:

Toss shrimp with garlic powder, paprika, lemon pepper, lemon juice, and olive oil.

Place the cooking tray in the air fryer basket.

Select Air Fry mode.

Set time to 8 minutes and temperature 400 F then press START.

The air fryer display will prompt you to ADD FOOD once the temperature is reached then add shrimp in the air fryer basket.

Shake basket halfway through.

Serve shrimp with lemon slices.

Baked Mahi-Mahi

Preparation Time: 10 minutes

Cooking Time: 12 minutes

Serve: 4

Ingredients:

4 Mahi Mahi fillets

1 tsp oregano

1 tsp garlic powder

3 tbsp olive oil

1 tsp cumin

1 tsp onion powder

1 tsp paprika

1/2 cayenne

1/2 tsp pepper

1/2 tsp salt

Directions:

Place fish fillets on the baking sheet and drizzle with oil.

In a small bowl, mix together cumin, onion powder, paprika, cayenne, oregano, garlic powder, pepper, and salt.

Rub fish fillets with a spice mixture.

Place the cooking tray in the air fryer basket.

Line air fryer basket with parchment paper.

Select Bake mode.

Set time to 12 minutes and temperature 400 F then press START.

The air fryer display will prompt you to ADD FOOD once the temperature is reached then place fish fillets onto the parchment paper in the air fryer basket.

Serve and enjoy.

Flavorful Prawns

Preparation Time: 10 minutes

Cooking Time: 6 minutes

Serve: 4

Ingredients:

12 prawns

1 tsp chili powder

1 tsp red chili flakes

1 tbsp vinegar

1 tbsp ketchup

3 tbsp mayonnaise

1/2 tsp sea salt

Directions:

In a bowl, toss prawns with chili flakes, chili powder, and salt.

Select Air Fry mode.

Set time to 6 minutes and temperature 350 F then press START.

The air fryer display will prompt you to ADD FOOD once the temperature is reached then place prawns in the air fryer basket.

In a small bowl, mix together mayonnaise, vinegar, and ketchup and serve with prawns.

Air Fry Blackened Shrimp

Preparation Time: 10 minutes

Cooking Time: 6 minutes

Serve: 4

Ingredients:

1 lb shrimp, peeled and deveined

1 tsp garlic powder

1 tsp onion powder

2 tbsp olive oil

2 tsp paprika

1/4 tsp cayenne

1 tsp dried oregano

Pepper

Salt

Directions:

In a bowl, toss shrimp with remaining ingredients.

Select Air Fry mode.

Set time to 6 minutes and temperature 400 F then press START.

The air fryer display will prompt you to ADD FOOD once the temperature is reached then place shrimp in the air fryer basket.

Serve and enjoy.

Jumbo Shrimp

Preparation Time: 10 minutes

Cooking Time: 6 minutes

Serve: 4

Ingredients:

1 lb jumbo shrimp

1 tsp steak seasoning

1/4 tsp crushed red pepper flakes

2 garlic cloves, minced

2 tsp olive oil

1 tbsp parsley, chopped

2 tsp lemon juice

1 tsp lemon zest

Directions:

In a bowl, toss shrimp with parsley, lemon juice, lemon zest, steak seasoning, red pepper flakes, garlic, and olive oil.

Select Air Fry mode.

Set time to 6 minutes and temperature 400 F then press START.

The air fryer display will prompt you to ADD FOOD once the temperature is reached then add shrimp in the air fryer basket.

Serve and enjoy.

Lemon Pepper White Fish

Preparation Time: 10 minutes

Cooking Time: 12 minutes

Serve: 2

Ingredients:

12 oz white fish fillets

1/2 tsp garlic powder

1/2 tsp onion powder

1/2 tsp lemon pepper seasoning

Pepper

Salt

Directions:

Spray fish fillets with cooking spray and season with onion powder, lemon pepper seasoning, garlic powder, pepper, and salt.

Select Air Fry mode.

Set time to 12 minutes and temperature 360 F then press START.

The air fryer display will prompt you to ADD FOOD once the temperature is reached then place fish fillets in the air fryer basket.

Serve and enjoy.

Italian Tilapia Fillets

Preparation Time: 10 minutes

Cooking Time: 17 minutes

Serve: 2

Ingredients:

1/2 lb tilapia fillets, remove bones

1/3 cup fresh parsley, chopped

1 tsp olive oil

1 tbsp garlic, minced

2 oz feta cheese, crumbled

2/3 cup tomatoes, chopped

Pepper

Salt

Directions:

In a medium bowl, mix together tomatoes, garlic, feta, parsley, and olive oil.

Spray tilapia fillets with cooking spray and season with pepper and salt.

Select Bake mode.

Set time to 17 minutes and temperature 400 F then press START.

The air fryer display will prompt you to ADD FOOD once the temperature is reached then place fish fillets in the air fryer basket and top with tomato mixture.

Serve and enjoy.

Greek Style Fish Fillets

Preparation Time: 10 minutes

Cooking Time: 10 minutes

Serve: 4

Ingredients:

24 oz salmon, cut into 4 pieces

1 tsp lemon zest

2 tbsp lemon juice

2 tbsp olive oil

1 tsp oregano

1 garlic clove, grated

1 tbsp yogurt

1/4 tsp pepper

1/4 tsp salt

Directions:

Add all ingredients except salmon in a baking dish and mix well.

Add salmon and coat well and let it sit for 30 minutes.

Select Bake mode.

Set time to 10 minutes and temperature 400 F then press START.

The air fryer display will prompt you to ADD FOOD once the temperature is reached then place the baking dish in the air fryer basket.

Serve and enjoy

Roasted Fish Fillets

Preparation Time: 10 minutes

Cooking Time: 15 minutes

Serve: 2

Ingredients:

1 lb red snapper fillet

1/4 tsp herb de Provence

1 garlic clove, crushed

2 tbsp olive oil

3/4 cup white wine

2 fresh rosemary sprigs

Pepper

Salt

Directions:

Season fish fillet with pepper and salt and place in baking dish.

Drizzle oil over fish.

Place rosemary, garlic, and herb de Provence on top of fish.

Select Roast mode.

Set time to 10 minutes and temperature 400 F then press START.

The air fryer display will prompt you to ADD FOOD once the temperature is reached then place the baking dish in the air fryer basket.

Pour wine over fish fillet and continue roast for 5 minutes.

Serve and enjoy.

Shrimp with Cherry Tomatoes

Preparation Time: 10 minutes

Cooking Time: 25 minutes

Serve: 4

Ingredients:

1 lb shrimp, peeled

1 tbsp garlic, sliced

2 cups cherry tomatoes

1 tbsp olive oil

Pepper

Salt

Directions:

Add shrimp, oil, garlic, tomatoes, pepper, and salt into the large bowl and toss well.

Transfer shrimp mixture into the baking dish.

Select Bake mode.

Set time to 25 minutes and temperature 400 F then press START.

The air fryer display will prompt you to ADD FOOD once the temperature is reached then place the baking dish in the air fryer basket.

Serve and enjoy.

Cod with Asparagus

Preparation Time: 10 minutes

Cooking Time: 20 minutes

Serve: 4

Ingredients:

1lb cod, cut into 4 pieces

1 leek, sliced

1 onion, quartered

2 tomatoes, halved

2 tbsp olive oil

1/2 tsp oregano

1/2 tsp red chili flakes

1/2 cup olives, chopped

8 asparagus spears

1/4 tsp pepper

1/4 tsp salt

Directions:

In a baking dish, place fish pieces, olives, asparagus, leek, onion, and tomatoes.

Season with oregano, chili flakes, pepper, and salt and drizzle with olive oil.

Select Bake mode.

Set time to 20 minutes and temperature 400 F then press START.

The air fryer display will prompt you to ADD FOOD once the temperature is reached then place the baking dish in the air fryer basket.

Serve and enjoy.

Pesto Fish Fillets

Preparation Time: 10 minutes

Cooking Time: 20 minutes

Serve: 2

Ingredients:

2 salmon fillets

1/4 cup parmesan cheese, grated

For pesto:

1/4 cup parmesan cheese, grated

1/4 cup pine nuts

1/4 cup olive oil

1 1/2 cups fresh basil leaves

2 garlic cloves, peeled and chopped

1/2 tsp pepper

1/2 tsp salt

Directions:

Add all pesto ingredients into the food processor and process until smooth.

Place salmon fillet in a baking dish and spread 2 tablespoons of the pesto on each salmon fillet.

Sprinkle grated cheese on top of the pesto.

Select Bake mode.

Set time to 20 minutes and temperature 400 F then press START.

The air fryer display will prompt you to ADD FOOD once the temperature is reached then place the baking dish in the air fryer basket.

Serve and enjoy.

Mediterranean Salmon

Preparation Time: 10 minutes

Cooking Time: 20 minutes

Serve: 1

Ingredients:

4 oz salmon fillet

1/2 lemon juice

1 garlic clove, sliced

1/4 onion, diced

5 grape tomatoes

1 tbsp fresh parsley, chopped

1 tbsp olive oil

Pepper

Salt

Directions:

Add all ingredients except lemon juice into the mixing bowl and let sit for one hour.

Select Bake mode.

Set time to 20 minutes and temperature 350 F then press START.

The air fryer display will prompt you to ADD FOOD once the temperature is reached then transfer bowl mixture in the air fryer basket.

Drizzle with lemon juice.

Serve and enjoy.

Salsa Fish Fillets

Preparation Time: 10 minutes

Cooking Time: 15 minutes

Serve: 4

Ingredients:

4 halibut fish fillets

2 tsp olive oil

3 tbsp fresh basil, chopped

2 tomatoes, chopped

2 garlic cloves, minced

1 tsp oregano, chopped

Directions:

In a bowl, mix together chopped tomatoes, garlic, oregano, and basil.

Arrange fish fillets in the baking dish and top with tomato mixture.

Select Bake mode.

Set time to 15 minutes and temperature 350 F then press START.

The air fryer display will prompt you to ADD FOOD once the temperature is reached then place the baking dish in the air fryer basket.

Serve and enjoy.

Lightning Source UK Ltd.
Milton Keynes UK
UKHW052325290421
382826UK00004B/24